Something Has To Change

Little Change – Big Results

By

Mark "Lefty" Holencik

www.7daymentaldiet.com

Author's Note

The information and recommendations presented in this book are based on the author's personal experience. The author of this book is not a doctor and does not dispense medical or prescribe the use or the discontinuance of any medications. This book is not intended to take the place of medical advice of your doctor. Application of the information and recommendations described herein are undertaken at the individual's own risk.

All the recommendations herein contained are made without guarantees on the part of the author, or the publisher, their agents, or employees. The author and publisher disclaim all liability in connection with the use of the information presented herein.

Table of Contents

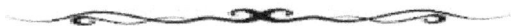

I would like to thank

Dr. Mike Murdock

for teaching me how to write a book. Without his guidance I would be carrying my story inside me.

My people are destroyed for a lack of knowledge.

Hosea 4:6

My Story

*Let your light shine before men
in such a way that they may see
your good works, and glorify
your Father who is in heaven.*

Matthew 5:16

Growing up I never remember my Grandfather being in the same day I was. Today I understand he had some form of dementia. As a child it was confusing, but it always stuck with me. I thought about it often through the years.

Knowing enough about heredity, my chances of landing up like this were good. Then looking at my other Grandfather, heart disease was also in my future.

If you looked at my lifestyle, you could not imagine that these things were on my mind and were of a real concern to me. For between the ages of 16 and 19, drinking and drugs were a constant part of my life. At 19, I put the drugs down. My diet was to eat whatever I pleased. Heartburn and memory loss were normal everyday occurrences. The two things that scared me the most, memory loss and feeling like I was having a heart attack, were my constant companions.

At the age of 35, I put down the drink. Memory loss and poor concentration was still there, but the heartburn was gone. I resigned myself to the fact that I may have not stopped in time. I was overweight from all the drinking. I weighed 210 pounds. Just from putting the drink down my weight dropped to 190 in 2 months. Over the next year I lost more weight and leveled off at 180-185.

Having a very physically demanding job allowed me to eat whatever I pleased in any quantities and not gain weight. So there was no need for me to change. I remember saying that all the taste of food was in the parts that were unhealthy and I would not change my diet till my life depended on it.

Luckily, this did not come to pass. I made the changes that needed to be made before my body showed the major signs of giving out.

Around the age of 50, I was doing less and less of the physical part of the job. It was a slow process when I put on weight and my waist went from 32" to 34" at the age of 55. If I gained one more ounce I would have need to go to a 36" waist. My weight was a constant thought. Every time I bent over or stood up I needed to pull my pants up. I could no longer move the way I used to.

Finally, arriving at the point where buying a pair of pants with a 36" waist was totally unacceptable to me. This coupled with my Grandfather's dementia, inspired me to make the commitment to myself to do what needed to be done.

Reflecting back to when I was 16, had a 32" waist and weighed 175 pounds, I set this as the goal. Looking through some old pictures, I found one of Bets and me at my goal weight. I made a Dream Board of my goals as an example. This picture of Bets and me was the center of the Dream Board.

The following month I was giving a retreat on The 7 Day Mental Diet. As part of my presentation on focusing the mind to achieve the goals you set for yourself, I knew that in using my own Dream Board as an example in this seminar, I was holding myself accountable to this group of 25 guys. Having people that you are accountable to increases your chance for success by 80%.

That was in March. The third weekend in May, I was at a weekend retreat. The one bathroom had a doctor's scale. Weighing myself, I was shocked. 218 pounds was hard to believe, but it gave me the final commitment and resolve to change my eating habits.

The first change was to drink more water. 2 weeks later I started to eat more fresh fruits and vegetables. In 10 weeks I had lost 30 pounds. The second week in August I was giving another seminar to the same group of guys. It felt good to be able to show that the Dream Board worked. The following March I was going to give another seminar to the same group. At that seminar, I had accomplished my goal of 175 pounds and a 32" waist.

We have a farmers market close to us. They are open year round. This is a blessing. I started to go there every Saturday afternoon near closing time. I found one stand that makes me feel special. When people make me feel special, I go back. I made my new life style a special event. The workers are calling out the specials of the hour. Sometimes when I walk in the building one of the workers will stop their calling and say, "I have an announcement, Lefty has just entered the building." I have made new friends. Events like this make me more determined to stay on this path. Even loners need this sense of belonging.

None of the weight I have lost was through exercise. This is not to brag, but to tell my story exactly as it has happened. I have made attempts to exercise and stopped.

You only fail when you quit. I will try until I succeed. I do not beat myself up. To beat myself up would ensure that I would stop the things that I am successful at. *Winners never quit, and quitters never win.* Keep up the fight. Never ever quit.

The rest of this book will be to tell you what I did and what I learned about weight-loss. I have not written this book as medical advice. Check with your doctor and tell him what you plan to do. You may need medical attention while losing weight. I am not a dietitian; I am only stating what I have done. Having a dietitian design a food plan will give you a balance of the vitamins and minerals you need to sustain a healthy lifestyle.

Why Most Diets Fail

The first to plead his case seems right, Until another comes and examines him.

Proverbs 18:17

Most diets address:

- The amount of food you eat.
- The kinds of food you eat.
- When you eat.
- Exercise

I have found that is to "Have the Cart Before the Horse". These things play a part in being healthy, but only a very small part in actual weight-loss. The amount of food you eat will cause you to lose weight, but as you know from experience it will come back sooner or later. You say that I have the "Cart Before the Horse"? How can that be?

Here is how it was explained to me.

1. How long can you go without food?
   Months.
2. How long can you go without water?
   Days
3. How long can you go without breathing?
   Minutes

Most diets address your food consumption and pay little attention to keeping you properly hydrated. Also I have never heard correct breathing addressed as a part of losing weight.

I have not lost any weight from exercising. At the time of this writing, I still am trying to overcome my mental block about exercise. I will overcome the block.

Since I started this journey by accident I have done weight-loss in the correct order. The main focus was to eat the proper foods to lower my risk of getting some form of dementia. I had seen too many people focused on food fail at dieting. The weight I was losing would not get me to my goal of not getting dementia. The amount of food I ate would take care of itself if my main focus was keeping my brain healthy and active.

At the age of 36 I had corrected my breathing patterns. Since then my diaphragm breathing has improved through practice.

I always drank a lot of water due to the demanding job I had as a roofer, but I increased the amount of water with the changes in the kinds of food I ate.

I made a decision to introduce fresh fruits and vegetables to my menu. I did not consciously eliminate foods from my diet in the beginning. It was only after 7 months and losing 35 pounds that I made the choice to eliminate certain foods from my diet. This was a healthy choice and not a weight-loss choice.

So while what you eat is important to healthy dieting, ultimately your long term weight-loss goals, like mine, depends on learning how to breathe properly and stay properly hydrated.

Proper Breathing

Feelings come and go like clouds in a windy sky. Conscious breathing is my anchor.

Thich Nhat Hanh

Years ago a mentor told me I did not know how to breathe; I told him he was crazy. Everyone knows how to breathe. If you did not know how to breathe you would die.

I have since learned that yes, we all breathe, just not properly. We breathe in a way that produces adrenaline, which increases stress. Stress is a big factor in weight gain. Besides, breathing is not only meant to keep us alive, but calm and healthy, not stressed.

How do you know if you are breathing correctly? Try this test.

Take a deep breath.

What expanded?

15

Was it your chest?

Was it your abdomen?

If the primary movement was in your chest, you are breathing incorrectly. Your abdomen should be expanding. This is called diaphragm breathing.

Breathing can be trained for both positive and negative influences on health. Chronic stress can lead to a restriction of the connective and muscular tissue in the chest resulting in a decrease range of motion of the chest wall. Due to more rapid, shallow breathing, the chest does not expand as much as it would with slower, deeper breaths. As a result much of the air exchange occurs at the top of the lung tissue towards the head.

In addition, the greatest amount of blood flow occurs in the lower lobes of the lungs. People that breathe from their chests with rapid, shallow breathes, limit the air expansion in these areas resulting in less oxygen transfer to the blood. This, in turn, causes a poor delivery of nutrients to the tissues. Finally, since oxygen along with water, also removes toxins from the blood, if you take in less oxygen your body is removing fewer toxins.

Your body to defend itself from these toxins makes fat cells. Fat is actually your body's defense system way of keeping you alive. It produces a fat cell that encapsulates the toxin. As you take in more water and oxygen your body begins to detoxify. Hence you lose weight.

The good news is that similar to learning to play a new game or tying your shoes, you can train your body to improve its breathing technique. With regular practice you will breathe from the abdomen most of the time, even while asleep.

My chest breathing was so ingrained that it took me awhile to just get my diaphragm to move. I tried for a couple of minutes for 3 or 4 days. Then finally, my diaphragm moved.

To practice breathing properly, follow these steps.

1. Lay on your back. If you are standing or sitting your stomach muscles are being used to hold you up straight. This makes it hard for you to train your diaphragm to breathe properly.
2. Place your hands on the abdomen. When you take a deep breath, your hands will start to rise.
3. After exhaling through the mouth, take a slow deep breath in through your nose and hold it for a count of 6. Do this as long as you are able. Your stamina will increase with time.
4. Slowly exhale through your mouth for a count of 8. As all the air is released without effort, contract your abdominal muscles to completely evacuate the remaining air from the lungs. It is important to remember that we deepen respirations not by inhaling more air but through completely exhaling it.
5. Repeat this cycle five more times for a total of 6 deep breaths and try to breathe at a rate of one breath every 10 seconds (or 6 breaths per minute). At this rate your heart rate variability increases which has a positive effect on cardiac health.

In general, exhalation should be twice as long as inhalation. The use of the hands on your abdomen is only needed to help you train your breathing. As you develop the ability to breathe into the abdomen, it is no longer needed.

Inhale through your nose.

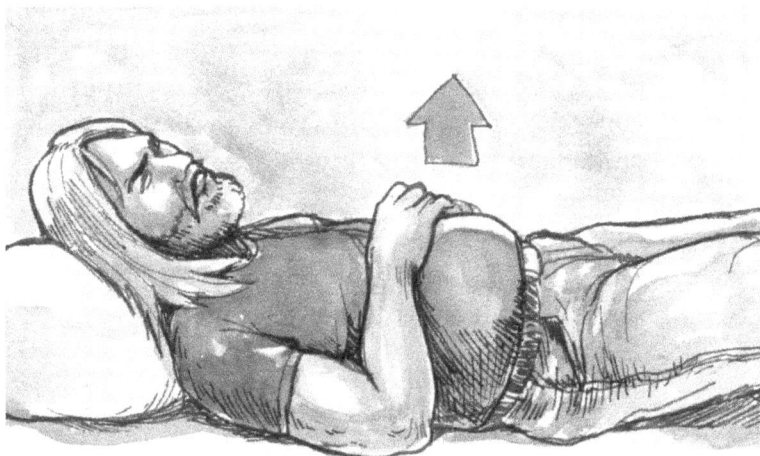

Exhale Through Your Mouth.

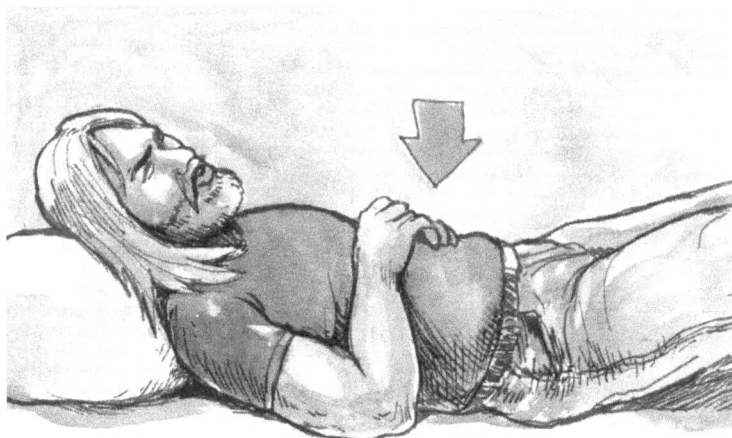

Abdominal breathing is just one of many breathing exercises. But it is the most important one to learn. The more it is practiced, the more natural it will become improving the body's internal rhythm.

Once you have trained yourself to breathe correctly you can add words or phrases that have meaning to you.

For example as you breathe in say

- **"In with the good"** on exhaling **"out with the bad"**.
- **"Breath is life"** on exhaling **"I am purifying my body"**.
- **"Relaxation"** on exhaling **"anger or stress"**

Use any words or phrases that make sense to you. While inhaling pick a word that will have a positive impact, and on the exhaling use a word that describes what you are trying to get rid of.

Proper breathing will relieve hunger pains. Breathing also cleanses the body of toxins.

- **Do not give up.**
- **Do not give up.**
- **Do not give up.**

Once you accomplish that, give yourself credit. It is a big deal. Make small achievable goals. Celebrate your accomplishments. Let go of the morbid reflecting. You only look at the past to learn from it. That is how to lead a successful life.

- **You did it!**
- **You did it!**
- **You did it!**

<u>Notes</u>

Proper Hydration

Water is the only drink for a wise man.

Henry David Thoreau

Dehydration is rampant in our society. It is said that 80% of the people are dehydrated. You probably think you are not dehydrated because you are not thirsty. Thirst in most people is a sign of *severe* dehydration. When the brain needs energy it sends signals for both food and water. We interpret these two signals as the one for food. This is partly because we are taught that energy comes from food. However, the body needs water also to be fully energized.

A reliable indicator of dehydration is the color of your urine. Clear or light-colored urine means you are well hydrated, whereas a dark yellow or amber color usually signals dehydration. So drink plenty of water! Soda, diet soda, coffee, and most of the fluids you drink will hydrate you because they have water in them; the problem however, is with the other ingredients in these beverages. Most non-water drinks have unhealthy ingredients. **They have harmful side-effects on your health.** Some ingredients, such as alcohol, caffeine, sugars, and dairy products actually cause dehydration. **These drinks actually call for your body to get rid of fluids to flush out the contents of the drinks.** The best thing we can use to hydrate ourselves is water.

It is important to know the common symptoms of dehydration, especially since some of them are often mistaken for other illnesses. People sometimes treat these symptoms with over the counter drugs or with prescriptions and this only exacerbates the problem. The real problem is a simple lack of water.

The bodies is made to heal itself. These side-effects may not show up for years. Only after all the reserves of the needed nutrients used to deal with these other ingredients are used up will this show. In our society we do not call them side-effects. We call them getting old or part of the aging process. This leaves us off the hook, and prevents us from making the changes we need to stay healthy.

It is important to know the common symptoms of dehydration and how they affect the body.

Symptoms of Dehydration

1. **Constipation**. When dehydrated, the colon removes more water than normal in order to provide fluid for other critical parts of the body.
2. **Fatigue**. Water is the single best source of energy in the human body. Fatigue is one of the earliest signs of dehydration.
3. **Joint problems**. Cartilage is mainly water. Dehydration weakens cartilage and delays repair.
4. **Digestive disorders**. Dehydration reduces the secretion of digestive juices and can also lead to acid reflux, ulcers and gastritis.
5. **Asthma and allergies.** A large amount of water evaporates during normal breathing. When dehydrated, the body attempts to reduce water loss by restricting airways.

6. **High blood pressure**. Blood is about 83% water. Dehydration causes blood to thicken, making it more difficult to pump throughout the body.
7. **Cholesterol**. Dehydration causes cellular water loss. The body produces more cholesterol in an attempt to stop cells from losing water.
8. **Weight gain**. Dehydration causes the body to store toxins in fat cells. The body will not release fat unless it is adequately hydrated to safely remove the toxins.
9. **Skin disorders**. The skin is the body's largest organ of elimination. Dehydration prevents the movement of toxins through the skin and causes premature wrinkling.
10. **Liver, kidney, bladder problems**. Dehydration increases the concentration of toxins that these organs must eliminate on a daily basis. The accumulation of toxic waste can cause infection, inflammation and pain.
11. **Lack of mental focus or concentration**. The brain is about 95% water. Thus, dehydration can significantly impair brain and nerve cell function, including loss of memory and concentration.
12. **Premature aging**. Dehydration accelerates the visible effects of aging skin as well as the withering and wrinkling effect on the internal organs.

This leads us to the question: how much water should we be drinking every day in order to maintain optimal health? To figure this out, take your weight and divide it in half. Then drink that amount in ounces each day. It is that simple—half your weight in ounces of water. Drinking water alone will start you on the journey of losing weight.

Prove it to yourself. Do not change your eating habits for a week, just hydrate yourself properly and see what happens.

The first day drink half your weight in ounces of water. The next day drink 8 ounces more. Stay with that amount or more for the rest of the week. Being properly hydrated will send a signal to the fat cells that the kidneys are now operating at full power and will be taking in more shipments of toxins. Your fat cells will start to send toxins back into the blood stream for elimination, and you will begin to lose weight. You will also have increased energy from the fat cells. Together these will naturally curb your appetite.

Spreading your water intake across your day is the best way to hydrate. Start your day before breakfast with 12 to 16 ounces of water. Do the same before each meal. Keep doing this and you will be amazed at the results.

Just remember:

Your body is 75% water. Dehydration occurs when there is not enough water to replace what is lost throughout the day.

Foods

And God said, Behold, I have given you every herb yielding seed, which is upon the face for all the earth, and every tree, in which is the fruit of a tree yielding seed, to you it shall be for food.

Genesis 1:29

Before I start this chapter on food, here is my disclaimer: What I am about to present to you is in no way a statement on what you need to do. It is only what I have done. Your choice of food needs to be enjoyable to you or you will quit at some point. You also need to introduce some foods that you do not like. Over time you will develop a taste for them. I am sharing my experiences with the hope it will inspire you to make the changes you need to make in your diet.

My journey of introducing fresh fruits and vegetables into my diet led me to our local farmers market. In fact, my weekly trips to the farmers market on Saturday afternoons have turned into fun social events. The more I travel through life the more I see you need to find new ways to make life more enjoyable, and for me discovering the people and fresh produce of a farmers market has brought me great joy.

Learning to eat fresh fruits and vegetables has taught me many things. One of the things I found out was that you cannot eat all the fresh food fast enough. It starts to spoil. Luckily new ideas come to me all the time. Why would they not come? We were born to create. So one day while thinking of the food I was throwing away, the thought crossed my mind: "You like trail mix, right Lefty? Why not dehydrate the food that is going to spoil and make your own trailmix?"

So the next step in my journey was to buy a dehydrator. Not only did this solve the wasting food problem, but the entire process of dehydrating has become a part of my spiritual life. The repetition of slicing everything so thinly and delicately has made the time I spend doing it into a way of meditating. It is a peaceful experience for me.

Over time this meditation has turned into dehydrating 50% of my diet. In fact, now I buy most of my food just to dehydrate it. This has completely solved the food spoiling issue since dehydrated foods don't spoil. I mix up a trail mix in a tupperware container and I'm good to go. No need to have a cooler for lunch. I like things simple.

I do not eat a lot of cooked foods anymore-- hardly any processed foods. Salads are easy to prepare, and since I enjoy dehydrating foods so much, and find them flavorful and interesting, I simply do not have a need or desire for cooked foods.

I have even stopped eating meat. This decision just seemed to naturally happen over time. Reading about the nutritional value of foods I found that meats take a lot of time and energy to digest. This tells me there are better foods to eat.

Another thing I discovered is that there is nothing good about dairy products. Man is the only species on earth that drinks milk after the age of 2. Every other species before the age of 2 switches to water. Even weirder yet is that we are the only creatures that drink milk from other animals!

That said, dairy products were the hardest thing for me to give up in my diet, and in particular, cheese. That was the really hard one. Giving up other dairy products was easy.

But I am glad I did.

I have always had to carry a hanky with me year round. My nose was always running or stuffed up. As soon as I stopped eating dairy products my nose cleared up. I have not used a hanky in 9 months, and I feel a lot better—more energy, more mental clarity.

So what do I eat if I no longer eat processed foods, dairy products or meat? Fruits and vegetables.

When deciding what vegetables to eat the rule of thumb is: eat the rainbow. When picking your vegetables for the week pick by color. The more colors you can eat the better your nutritional needs will be met. Each color provides a different need for your body.

Fruits are the closest foods to usable nutrition. This means they take very little energy to digest. Within a half an hour fruit has moved through your stomach. They also have a lot of protein. Vegetables take a little more energy to digest, but not much. They too move quickly through your body.

I did not need scientific studies to discover that fruits and vegetables move through my body more quickly. Since drinking enough water and eating fruits, vegetables, and nuts, I began moving my bowels at least 3 times a day compared to what I used to...

Initially this scared me. I thought that I was getting sick or had diarrhea, but then the thought came to me that dogs do their duty a half hour after eating. Maybe this is the way it is supposed to be. I found out that this is true for dogs as well as humans.

Another confusing thing for me when I started eating only raw foods was it seemed to me that not only was I moving my bowels more, but the volume of those movements increased. It turns out that the toxins stored in my fat cells were being excreted, making it natural to have higher volume bowel movements.

I share these personal experiences so you know if they start happening to you, it's OK. The main thing is that when I started eating raw foods, my body changed. It changed for the better. I had more energy, more mental clarity, and I realized that my goals of living a healthier, longer life were being achieved. I knew I was helping my body and my brain. I was becoming more and more the person I wanted to become.

For the LORD your God is bringing you into a good land—a land with brooks, streams, and deep springs gushing out into the valleys and hills; ⁸ a land with wheat and barley, vines and fig trees, pomegranates, olive oil and honey

Deuteronomy 8:7-8

<u>Notes</u>

Proper PH Level

Be not among winebibbers,
Among gluttonous eaters of flesh

Proverbs 23:20

The purpose of this brief chapter is to
introduce you to the subject of PH levels.
It is a basic explanation meant to just get
you started on your journey. It is
important however to the success of
gaining long term weight loss. Just as a
swimming pool needs regular monitoring
to be safe to swim in, your body needs the
blood stream to have a safe PH level to
live a long healthy life.

The blood's PH is measured on a scale of
1-14, 1 being totally acidic and 14 being
totally alkaline. The perfect balance is
7.36, tilting the scales a little towards
alkaline. You need both acid and alkaline
for your body to function properly. The
more control you have over your intake of
each, the more control you have over your
health.

Your stomach needs to be more acidic then the rest of your body. The extra acid in your stomach is to break down the food you eat into a usable form. Acid is also needed to keep the electrical currents in your body flowing. But if you have more then is needed, it starts to break down your body tissue.

Just like fat cells protect you from toxins in your body from killing you, cholesterol keeps acid from breaking down the walls of your blood vessels. If the blood vessels have holes in them from acid eating through them you will die. Keep your acid levels where they need to be and your body will not make cholesterol to line your blood vessels. Over time your blood vessels will clean themselves out just like the fat cells will when you are properly hydrated.

When you are too acidic the body needs to protect itself. Toxins in the bloodstream are taken to the lungs, kidneys, liver and skin to expel them. Dehydration lowers the kidneys' effectiveness. This causes waste to stay in the blood waiting for the lungs, liver and skin to remove them. As you keep adding more acidic food to your body, the blood is polluted to dangerous levels. Luckily, the body is an amazing machine and will do anything it can to preserve your life. In its efforts to keep you alive and healthy, your brain sends a message to take some of the toxins out of your blood and encapsulate them in fat cells. Fat is really your body protecting itself from certain death.

Just imagine the garbage trucks coming through your neighborhood. When they are full they go to the landfill to unload. The landfill is running behind. They can not unload the trucks as fast as they arrive. What do the garbage trucks do? They will sit there and wait. The garbage continues to ferment becoming more toxic. Some of the trucks decide to look for another place to dump their load. The truck finds a place but it says "No Dumping". The driver must pick up the rest of his garbage. So he dumps his load anyway. The place the load was dumped was the skin. The toxins come out of the skin. We call it acne among a host of other skin ailments. Another truck finds a spot, but there is a sign that says "No

Dumping". He also needs to get rid of his load to finish his neighborhood. He dumps his load and the nose starts to run and gets clogged up. This keeps happening throughout the body. The toxins must come out or eat away at the body.

The crazy thing is when the skin starts to push these toxins out the body and the nose starts running, the lungs start to cough... What do we do? We run to the drug store. We buy creams and ointments to push the toxins back in so we do not have acne. We buy drugs to dry up the nose so the toxins stay in the body. We buy medicine so we do not cough. We try to stop the body from purifying itself.

Eventually the body cannot hold up and we get sick and die. You can prevent this. Pay attention to what you eat and drink. If you only use taste as the factor in deciding what you eat, somewhere along the line you will pay the price for your decisions.

Here is a list to get you familiar with the more acidic foods.

Fruits

Currants, blueberries, cranberries, canned fruits and glazed fruits are all examples of fruits that are acidic. The canned and glazed versions are acidic because they have sweeteners and preservatives added. Processed fruit juices are also high in acidity.

Grains

Processed grains and baked goods that are made with them are high in acidity. Examples of these include white bread, white rice, pasta, biscuits, bagels, doughnuts, pastries and crackers. These are also low in fiber and nutrients.

Dairy Products

All forms of milk, yogurt, cream cheese, cottage cheese, butter, ice cream and hard cheese are all high in acid. This goes for the non-fat versions all the way up to the whole-fat versions. Eggs are also high in acid.

Meats and Fish

Processed meats like bacon, sausage, ham and corned beef are all high in acid. Chicken, turkey, red meat, shellfish, seafood, lamb, organ meats, pork and game meats are also high in acid. Shellfish, seafood and game meats are the lowest in fat out of all of these.

Nuts and Oils

Nuts that are high in acid include pecans, walnuts, peanuts, cashews and pistachios. This also includes the butters that are made from them. Oils that are high in acid include olive, sesame, safflower, sunflower, avocado, corn and canola oil.

Beverages

All forms of alcohol are high in acid no matter whether they are light or low in calories. Examples of these include beer, wine, hard liquor, spirits and scotch. Other beverages that are high in acid include soda, coffee, black tea and cocoa.

As you can see, processing foods raises acid levels. Whole foods are the best foods to eat.

In addition to the types of foods you eat, emotions play a big role in ph levels. We all know the effects of anger on health. Anger and its bedfellow, stress, both make the body more acidic.

How can you help make your body more alkaline? One way is to reduce stress in your life and to find healthy ways to process your anger. The easiest ways however to make your body more alkaline are to eat more green vegetables and drink more water. I also drink a green drink through out the day consisting of powered wheat grass, various vegetables, barley grass, and so on. Green drinks add plenty of alkaline to your system. Since my green drink is in a powder form, I can take it anywhere I go and add it to my water. I always have plenty of energy and always stay hydrated and my green drinks are a big reason why.

The best green drink I have found comes from a company called Amazing Grass. Its ingredients are pure and natural—one of the best on the market.

The more control you have over your diet, the more control you have over your health. Most of the diseases we have today are caused by our lifestyle. Obesity, heart disease, cancer and anxiety disorders can be controlled or eliminated by diet.

People, Places and Things

If anyone does not obey our instruction in this letter, take special note of that person and do not associate with him

Thessalonians 3:14

"Birds of a feather flock together."

This is so true. If you are going to make lasting changes in your life you will need to take a look at your environment.

Work, friends, and family all play a part in who we are. They fill a need inside each of us. They help us find social fulfillment in varying degrees. Even if they have negative effects on us, we still get a sense of belonging from them. This need for belonging is so strong that we sometimes overlook unhealthy behaviors to fill this need in us.

This is called "Social Proofing". Social Proofing is when we start to gather facts to make a decision then use our social circles to finalize the decision. We use their behaviors as facts. Everyone else is doing it so it must be right.

The groups mentioned—coworkers, family, and friends, have unspoken rules for membership. Deciding to lose weight and live a healthy lifestyle, may go against these rules. Keep in mind however, that these are the same influences that made it okay to gain weight in the first place. They may not make it okay to lose weight even if you are the only one that is overweight in your group. Therefore, they will try to force or coerce us into giving up and getting back in step with the way things always were.

When I decided to change my life, I went through this with most of the people I knew. They made fun of my new lifestyle in both subtle and not so subtle ways. I decided not to talk about the changes I was making to my eating habits, with these people other than to just acknowledge that I was, in fact, making changes. It was easier for both sides. The ones that would have me remain the same did not want to think about their own eating habits, and my talking about what I was doing was taken as a judgment on them. These were things they did not want to face in themselves.

Other times when trying to have conversations about health with people, who did not want to change, they would only want to talk about the negative side-effects of their lifestyle, but rarely the solution to them. They would not want to complete the conversation with how to reverse the downward trends in their health. They would sum up our conversations about health with: "Oh well, we are just getting older." In other words they were saying: "This conversation is over. Leave this subject alone. I am not going to change."

I personally refuse to believe I am too old to change. So here again, to control the negative input from others on this subject, I simply limit whom I talk to about my

health and how I am trying to live as long
as possible and be active and alert till the
day I die.

If you experience similar social issues with
the people in your life, ask yourself: Are
you willing to make new friends with
people who live the new way you are
trying to live? I did. These social factors
are huge. But you are worth it.

Exercise

A good plan executed today is better than a perfect plan executed at some indefinite point in the future.

George S. Patton

I struggle with exercise. I have maintained the weight loss of 48 lbs. without exercising. My job is no longer very physical. Intellectually I know that exercise is crucial to my long term health. I still am fairly active and keep my body moving. I need to win this battle and I will.

Here is where the trouble lies with all progress, the internal battle with you. You desire a change because intellectually you know the change would be good for you. And yet even though you feel the effects of not implementing the change, you rationalize keeping the status quo. We are too quick to call it being lazy. But, when we look at the rest of our lives, to say we are lazy is ridiculous. Looking at all our past accomplishments big or small, and our daily routine, this does not fit the definition of laziness. We are strong determined people. Most times we do not even resort to prayer to accomplish our goal. We just get it done. We look at the task and say "I did that before. I can do it again." Or, "I did something similar and I can adapt."

I was conditioned to see myself as lazy by well meaning adults. There is no way to know how a person will process the things we are told as a child. The message will motivate some and cripple others. We may also have a mixture of the two. We might find something we want to accomplish and even get it done and yet still have the feeling of being a failure. We pick apart the success not based on the accomplishment itself, but on all the little trivial things that did not ultimately keep us from our goal but that didn't go as we planned. These things *are* trivial. They did not stop us from reaching our goal. This is obvious to other people. But we focus on these things and so even though we may have accomplished something wonderful we still carry feelings of being failures. When other people try to tell us we did it, we cannot accept their praise and explain to them all these things that went wrong or are still wrong.

Always remember what Thomas Edison said when asked by a reporter ""How did it feel to fail 10,000 times before inventing the light bulb"? Edison said "I never failed once. I found 10,000 things that did not work and then I invented the light bulb".

We must remember this every time we do not reach our desired result. Start looking for a new approach to the goal.

Never ever give up.

Never ever give up.

Never ever give up.

It is helpful to see where we got the message of failure. It does not matter if it was as a child or as an adult. Just seeing and acknowledging the message as a lie will give you ammunition to wage a war against this message that seems to be our core truth.

Television may have been the primary place that gave us so many mixed messages. While watching sporting events and dreaming of being fit and healthy, we are being sold potato chips, beer, and recliners. Turning off the television is the first step in any exercise program. Turn off the phone when eating or exercising. We do not need the negative input from the television. Today it can also be from our smart phones. Put your smart phones to good use. Listen to motivational talks. Listen to audio books. I have lots of seminars on my phone. I am always teaching myself something when what I am doing does not need my total attention. Even if I cannot totally listen to what is being said my mind will still hear it. I listen to set of positive affirmations. You can download the affirmations from my website. blog.7daymentaldiet.net.

Seeing the truth will give you a new drive with the next attempt. Push yourself toward a goal you can accomplish. Celebrate crossing the goal line. Then pick a new goal and set out a course to achieving it.

So what about me and exercising? Here's my plan. What I am going to do right now is scary, for to put this in print is to convict myself.

I have been wrestling with how to start exercising. The thought has been to do 50 deep knee bends, 50 sit-ups, and 50 push-ups. Sitting here typing I just cannot see this plan coming to fruition. I need to say something here and it will be for all time. My mind keeps saying you can do 10 of each. Anyone can do 10. Yes, but will you stick to it? You have never stuck to exercising before. What will the people reading think about my first idea of starting at 50 and yet settling for 10? As I am writing this out the thought came to me: They are in the same boat or they would not be reading this book. They will be cheering for you to do 10. They will be saying "Do it, Go for it, you can do it". Thank You for the encouragement and the vote of confidence in me, but the voice of doubt will not stop: "But what if you fail and do not continue? It is inevitable that you will meet some of the readers either through the mail or face to face and they will ask. "Did you get to 50?" You may have to tell them 10 is all you can do consistently. Or worse yet, "No I have not even stayed with doing 10." They may have been doing well and this statement may cause *them* to quit.

One thing is for sure. I may not follow all the way through with getting to the goal of 50 or even doing 10 every day, but the thought to eliminate this from the book has not entered the discussion I am having with myself.

That shows how far I have come with the "Oh-So-Important Battle with Self-Talk." 20 years ago for sure my answer would have been just take this conversation out of the book. 5 years ago, 3 maybe, even 2, but no more. Who I am is who I am. That is all I have to work with. And if I share my inner struggles openly perhaps you will see you're not alone.

I have found a strength in my God, through sharing my weaknesses with others along the way. Here I am again with all this knowledge and experience, still not able to exercise on my own. Prayer always works, but it is the last place we go. *The conversation with myself continues.*

Get up and start now!

Get up and start now!

Get up and start now!

OKAY!

OKAY!

OKAY!

Okay
Already.

I will do
it.

Done!

I did
it!

Wow!

I am not
lazy!

"You are lazy," was the thought that came when I was contemplating doing 50 of each and then reduced it to 10. "Wimp" even came into my internal conversation. But I called the bluff on the fear of starting. By doing that, I learned a few things. First, the inner voice that told me to reduce the amount to 10 was not the voice of laziness. It was the all-knowing voice of my intuition that guides me. That voice was my God telling me "You are not ready to do 50. If you try 50 you will fail, and I do not want to see you fail. Try 10, you can do 10 and be a success." God told me "I like hanging out with winners". I am a winner. I did 10 of each.

When I got up to start the first thought was about which exercise I should do first. Knee bends are the easiest so maybe I should get the sit-ups out of the way. No, do the knee bends. Start with a success. First knee bends. But when I got down, I needed to balance myself. Failure! No, not failure. You just needed to balance yourself. So I balanced myself on all 10. Push-ups next, 2 sets of 5. I barely got the second set of 5 push-ups done. I knew that the sit-ups were not going to be easy. I thought "Well just do 1 or 2. At least you started, that in itself is a success. There is no failure here. Not starting is the failure." I did one. That took everything I had. Quit? No. You would have to get up and write that you could not do 10. Okay, maybe I can do two more. I did two more. They were a little easier than the first one. Maybe I can do ten? It would be nice to do ten and get up to complete this part of the book and say I did what I said I was going to do.

The waters will not part until you step into the River Jordan. You can stand there and wait till hell freezes over and the waters will not part till you step in.

When you bake a cake, some ingredients are for taste. Others are for texture. If you leave out some ingredients the cake will not turn out the way that you expect. Changing some ingredients will only change the taste. Changing other ingredients will cause the cake to flop.

If you want to have the success your mentor has follow the directions exactly.

Success feels good!

Success feels good!

Success feels good!

I compared myself to myself and came out a success. If I would have compared myself to someone else I would have failed.

My prayer is that I continue to do ten. When we meet I can say I am doing it. Ten seems like a lot right now. My goal is that I can proudly say I am doing more than ten, but this is a good place to start.

Using a Mentor

Mentorship is learning through the pain of another. Your future is determined by who you choose to believe.

Mike Murdock

Finding a mentor to help guide you is a very important part of the journey. If you can do it alone more power to you, but most people need a detached person to help them see all the sides of a certain situation. Hiring a mentor to help you do this is money well spent.

What is the difference between a friend and a mentor?

A friend accepts you the way you are.

A mentor does not accept you the way you are. A mentor sees you at the goal you set for yourself and always give you direction on how to get there. A mentor's strength and belief in you is a priceless asset to have on your side.

If you are planning on making these changes with a friend for support, still get a mentor. Depending on your friend to be strong when you are weak, and you being strong when they are weak, is risky. If you really want an objective guide on your journey to fulfilling your goals then having a mentor is a really good idea. Relying solely on friends, who may end up needing you more than you need them, is risky. Do you really want to take the chance of failing again?

So I say again,

Get a mentor.

My first mentor was a man named John. He gave me odd things to do that didn't seem related to my goals. This caused great mental battles with myself. Some of the things that he said to do did not make sense. I could not see how these tasks were going to help me reach my goal.

One of the things John told me to do was get a library card. I said "I do not need a library card". He said, "Okay". This was not the response I expected. I expected him to try and convince me that I should get the card. But he did not. This built a lot of trust with me. I could not manipulate him. He was not going to waste his time. He gave me direction and it was up to me to follow it or not. I got the message that what I did was not going to affect his life one way or the other.

The funny thing is when I made the decision to get the library card I thought it was going to be an easy thing to do. It was not. I remember just getting up and walking to the door of my home. I got to the door and looked outside and said, "I am not getting a library card." And then I sat back down. Even though my struggle to get a library card may sound silly, it really wasn't about the card. It was about following directions I didn't understand. I struggled with this for a few days, and then finally made it to my truck. When I got in my truck the same thought came: "You do not need a library card". After a few days of this, I started to drive to the library, each day making it a little closer. One day I found myself in the library parking lot, but I could not get out of the truck. So I left. The next day I went to a different library and still could not get out of the truck. I went to 3 different libraries before I went inside. Then it took a couple of times till I made it to the desk and applied for a card.

The mental battles that went on over the course of the weeks it took me to accomplish this were excruciating. But I did not quit. I knew I was the only one who was going to pay the price if I quit. John's life would go on as usual no matter what I did.

When I got the card I went to see John to let him know I had completed the task he had given me. He smiled with a mischievous grin and said "Now get a book on listening, because you do not know how to listen".

I would like to say I ran to the library and got a book on listening, but I did not. I did try. I was in the library standing in front of the books on listening. There were only 5 or 6 to choose from. I glanced through them. I looked at the few books on the subject and looked around at what were probably 50,000 books and decided that if this was an important topic there would be more books on the subject. So I went to another section and got a biography.

There are plenty of biographies to choose from. Again, I used "Social Proofing" to make my decision.

It took another couple of weeks till I surrendered and got a book on listening. It is one of the most important books I have ever read. The art of listening was very important to my future accomplishments.

Over time the battles have lessened. Now I will take direction that is given to me. I still have to struggle with a few things, but most of the time I put the direction I get into practice right away.

Experience has taught me that I have blind spots and cannot always see what is the best way to go. A mentor can see the blind spots and help guide me through them.

Having a mentor to keep me accountable is also invaluable. For without this system of accountability, I would not make the changes I need to as quickly as I do. If I ever make them.

I value my time today, and using a mentor is the best use of my time. He keeps me accountable. He gives me insights that would take me a lot of trial and error to see. Together we set goals and the times to complete these goals. I usually complete the goals in the times we set. If not, we evaluate our plan, look for any weaknesses, and then find new ways to achieve the goals.

The cost of using a mentor will easily pay for itself in the strides you will make in your life. Every great person who accomplishes great things has a mentor.

I am available for mentoring. If you are interested. You can contact me at lefty@7daymentaldiet.net.

A mentor is someone who sees more talent and ability within you, than you see in yourself, and helps bring it out of you.

Bob Proctor

<u>Notes</u>

Setting Your Goals

Our plans miscarry because they have no aim. When a man does not know what harbor he is making for, no wind is the right wind.

Lucius Seneca

Hopefully by reading this book you have acquired a greater desire and confidence that you can accomplish your healthy weight and size. The clearer you are about your dreams and goals the easier it is to get there.

1. Be specific with your goals. "I will lose weight" is not specific. "I will lose 25 pounds" is specific.

2. Give yourself a completion date. This needs to be 1 year or less. Goals over a year need to be broken down into smaller goals. If you plan on losing 200 pounds set a goal that you will accomplish in the next 6 months or a year. If you lose it all in a year, that would be a bonus.

3. Make sure your goals are realistic in the time you have set.

4. Find a mentor and discuss your goals with him or her. Always have an objective voice to help guide you.

Let us take some time right here and now to write down some of your goals and the time in which you would like to accomplish them. Ask yourself the following questions:

- What is your goal weight?
- What is your goal pants size?
- What cloths are you going to wear?

Once you can answer these questions clearly you have increased your chances of success dramatically.

Having a vision of how the quality of your life will improve once you lose your goal weight, will help you to stay focused and achieve your goal weight.

Here is a list of a well rounded purposeful life.

- Home - family, house and hobbies

- Business – your job or your own business
- Financial – savings, retirement, investments, loans
- Health – Overall health, diet, exercise...
- Charity – donating money, time and skills.
- Community – friends, church, and politics.

Now that you have set your goals, let's make them concrete. Go buy the pants or dress you are planning to wear. Get a calendar and circle the date. If you have a picture of you at your desired weight, put this picture someplace that you will see it regularly. Carry it with you. Impress this picture on your subconscious.

Find a person you are making yourself accountable to and let them know what your plans are. This person may be trying to lose weight too. If they are trying to lose weight too, this will be an added benefit. The important thing is they need to keep you accountable without using guilt.

The plans of the diligent lead surely to abundance, but everyone who is hasty comes only to poverty"

Proverbs 21:5

<u>Notes</u>

Telling Your Story

And he did not permit him but said to him, "Go home to your friends and tell them how much the Lord has done for you, and how he has had mercy on you.

Mark 5:19

Document your journey with pictures and words. This will help you get through the hard times. We all have a book inside us. When you get to your goal you can use your personal story to write your book. The world needs to hear your success story.

If I had known I was going to write a book, I would have taken pictures and kept a journal. When I decided to write this book, I needed to put my timeline together from memory. This is the hardest way to do things. One thing that helped me was from the beginning I started to share my story with anyone who showed an interest in losing weight. This helped me remember most of my experiences.

Make it easy on yourself and journal your progress along the way to your goal. The mental struggles that you have are important to document. The ups and downs are important to remember. Everyday is a new "before and after" picture.

Start to tell your ongoing story today. This will be a very important part of your success.

What do I mean by pictures?

- Find a picture of you when you were at your goal size/weight.
- Take a picture of yourself now.
- Take pictures of yourself along the way.
- Journal your hurdles
- Journal your mentor's suggestions and your reactions to them
- Journal your frustrations
- Journal your successes
- Journal your revelations

I make use of white boards to write things out. What I use for my white boards is a smooth white paneling you can find at any home center. It only costs around $15 for a 4' x 8' sheet. I panel the whole wall with it. You can get screws that have a chrome washer. This gives a finished look to the paneling and is easy to remove and replace with a new piece when the finish begins to wear. A 12' wall, 8' high will cost you around $70 and a little bit of time. But it's time and money well spent. It is easy to stand up and write on the wall when things come to mind. You can see the story coming together. When you want to move something you just write it somewhere else on the white board and erase it. This makes editing and gathering your thoughts and ideas very easy to do.

When I am on the phone talking it comes in handy too. I just write down any notes on the wall as I am talking. They are easy to see and find when they are written on the wall at eye level. White boards are a handy tool that can help make you very productive.

There is no agony like bearing an untold story inside of you.

Maya Angelou

The story was the bushman's
most sacred possession. These
people knew what we do not;
that without a story you have not
got a nation, or culture, or
civilization. Without a story of
your own, you haven't got a life
of your own.

Laurens Van der Post

Conclusion

Keep away from people who try to belittle your ambitions. Small people always do that, but the really great make you feel that you too, can become great.

Mark Twain

Write out your life like I did in the first chapter of this book. It must be written down. There is a magic that happens when you write things down. Find safe people to talk to. The sense of community in us must be fulfilled or we will fail. Birds of a feather flock together. There is a reason for this. There is safety in numbers. Proverbs tells us "Iron Sharpens Iron".

Visualizing where you are going is a valuable tool.

Make a dream board and keep it where you can see it. Constantly seeing what you want to do with your life will keep you emotionally involved with your goals. It will also reprogram your subconscious mind.

Weight-loss needs a holistic approach to succeed long term. The three main things in a holistic weight-loss program that determine success are

1. Breathing

2. Hydration

3. The Food You Eat

Remember these seven keys to success:

1. Educate yourself. Learning always makes change easier to stay committed to the goal. Ignorance makes it easier to quit and give up. Make a decision to do something every day to educate yourself.

2. Get a mentor. The time saved on making mistakes and quitting and starting over is well worth the money spent.

3. Stop treating dehydration with medication. Treat dehydration with water.

4. Listen to your body. Although you are making a conscious decision to change how much or what you are eating, a natural process will start to take place inside you. You will intuitively start to eat less. Also what you are eating will change naturally. You will lose the taste for certain foods that are not healthy. Listen to your body and your new diet will not be such a chore.

5. Affirm yourself. Every day read why you have made the goals you have chosen. This will help keep you focused on your goals.

6. Remember the "Tortoise and the Hare". *Slow and steady wins the race.* Sprinters are good for short distances. Permanent weight loss is not a sprinter's game. Develop a long distance strategy for your weight loss goal.

7. Find safe people to share your dreams with. Have meaningful conversations. Chit-chatting will leave you unfulfilled. And we all need to be filled with a sense of community. If it is not filled with meaningful relationships, food will be used to fill this need.

This book is only a beginning. Write to me and tell me about your success and trials. And if you cannot find a safe group of people to confide in then write to me. I may be able to put you in a group of like-minded people.

A journey of a thousand miles begins with a single step.

Lao-tzu

Again I say unto you, that if two of you shall agree on earth as touching anything that they shall ask, it shall be done for them of my Father who is in heaven.

Matthew 18:19

Questions or Mentoring contact me at:

lefty@7daymentaldiet.net

www.7daymentaldiet.com

www.ingramcontent.com/pod-product-compliance
Lightning Source LLC
Chambersburg PA
CBHW070911280326
41934CB00008B/1675